## *Praise for Write* ...
## *Journal Your* ...

*Write Your Self Well...Journal Your Self to Health*, by Ina Albert and Zoe Keithley, is a fresh workbook that should appeal to people who are looking for a way to deal with health problems. The authors do a masterful job of setting up a series of writing exercises that should be both fun and thought provoking. For the last twenty years, studies have been finding that expressive writing can boost physical and mental health. This workbook translates these research findings into action. This is an excellent journal.

James W. Pennebaker, Ph.D., Professor of Psychology
The University of Texas at Austin
Author of *Opening Up: The Healing Power of Expressing Emotions*

*Write Your Self Well...Journal Your Self to Health* is one of the best things I have read on the use of journaling to improve a patient's health. The objective of this work is to offer the benefits of expressive writing experienced by participants in twenty-plus years of clinical trials to all patients suffering from chronic or acute illness.

Leland R. Kaiser, Ph.D.
Futurist, Educator, Consultant, and Founder,
Kaiser Companies

A new book by Ina Albert and Zoe Keithley, *Write Your Self Well*, is a marvelous tutorial on the emotional and medical benefits of expressive writing. It emphasizes the healing benefits of journaling and offers directions that patients can take even if they've had no past writing experience. Journaling is a very important adjunctive therapy and the medical profession would do well to accept this new concept of self-help.

Wallace Salzman, MD
Author of the trilogy *Ortho-Para Novel/Treatises*


All too often, when sickness or age overtakes us, it begins to control us and define how we see ourselves. But we are not our sickness or the candles on the cake. We are always so much more. The wisdom found within the pages and exercises of *Write Your Self Well* will give you the skills to continue being a spirit-driven person. And when we are in touch with our spirit, even when the body weakens with age, sickness or handicap, we can do amazing things and continue to be unbelievably well and alive! Write your self well with these pages and you will discover how alive you really are!

Rev. John C. Cusick
Director, Young Adult Ministry Office
Archdiocese of Chicago

Patients and healthcare professionals working together toward healing is a concept that works. *Write Your Self Well...Journal Your Self to Health*, by Ina Albert and Zoe Keithley, is one of the best tools I've seen for facilitating that partnership. This journal can help transform normally passive patients into active partners in health by simply connecting them with their greatest loves and their deepest fears, all at the same time. This is a great idea!

Jim Schulman, Communication Consultant
and Body-Mind Therapist

# Write Your Self Well...

## Journal Your Self to Health

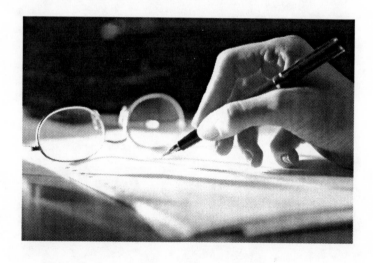

### By Ina Albert and Zoe Keithley

"Can you cure me, Doctor?"

*"I can diagnose and prescribe for you.*

*I can treat and counsel you."*

"But, will I feel whole again?

Will my spirit be renewed?"

*"Ah, that's your part of the job!"*

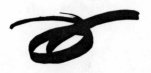

This book is designed to provide information and to encourage self-expression and self-understanding. Instructions and examples in this journal are provided for personal, private, educational and informational purposes only and do not constitute recommendations or instructions that might contradict or countermand those of patients' physicians or other healthcare professionals. Nor is it our purpose to provide psychological or professional services through this journal. If needed, patients should always first seek advice and services from competent professionals. The authors and Mountain Greenery Press will have neither liability nor responsibility to any person or entity with respect to any loss or damage caused, or alleged to be caused, directly or indirectly, by the information in this book.

Mountain Greenery Press
955 Northwoods Drive
Whitefish, MT 59937
(406) 863-2333

Library of Congress Control Number: 2004103478
ISBN: 0-9753196-0-4

Cover design: Andra Keller, Rocks-DeHart Public Relations

Printed in the United States of America

# Write Your Self Well...
## Journal Your Self to Health

# CONTENTS

# DEDICATION

This book is dedicated to you and your healing journey.

# ACKNOWLEDGMENTS

Over many years, we have come to appreciate both a patient's need to relate to healthcare professionals and a caregiver's need to feel valued by patients. Both need a stronger voice in the treatment process and both profit from being in a healing relationship with one another. We are grateful to the clinical and administrative professionals who have worked long and hard to make patient-centered and relationship-centered care a reality; to Fetzer Institute and The Planetree Alliance for showing us what it looks like to design and implement systems that put patients at the center of healthcare; and to Dr. Leland Kaiser for his brilliance, courage and encouragement to all of us throughout the years. All three have contributed inspiration and leadership to the development of healing environments and are thus responsible in large measure for creating this journal.

Our work stands on the shoulders of James Pennebaker, Ph.D., Professor of Psychology, The University of Texas at

Austin, whose pioneering research in the field of disclosure and expressive writing is the bedrock of this book. Our work is also grounded in the work of John Schultz, the creator of the Story Workshop® approach, Columbia College, and president of the Story Workshop Institute, both in Chicago, whose teaching methods inspired us to create the images used in this journal and pave the way for patients to move into written expression. We are indebted to behavioral psychologist Allan T. Paivio, Ph.D., Professor Emeritus, University of Windsor, Ontario, Canada, whose theories on the functioning of language are crucial to *Write Your Self Well...Journal Your Self to Health.*

The friends and mentors who have contributed their time, support and critique to this work begin with tough critic Adam Rose, who has given us much encouragement. A heartfelt thanks to author Jerry DeJaager for his patient coaching, advice and friendship through the past two years and to therapist and teacher Jim Schulman for his astute editing of the images included in our work. Many thanks to Bette BonFleur, co-founder of Ivanhoe, Inc. and Medical Breakthroughs television and internet health programming, for believing in us and in the healing value of journaling. Special thanks to medical writer

Don Radcliffe, to Richard Stone, founder of Storywork Institute, to GreystoneInteractive president, Kristine Peterson and to Celia Rocks of Rocks-DeHart Public Relations for believing in the unique value of *Write Your Self Well* and pushing us to move forward.

We are grateful for the encouragement of the Glacier Medical Group physicians in Whitefish, MT, for testing the journal with their patients. In particular, we want to thank Drs. Charles Charman and Suzanne Daniell for believing in the power of self-expression and for their commitment to seeing the health care experience through their patients' eyes and listening to their voices.

Most important kudos go to Rabbi Allen Secher, Ina's husband, partner and friend. He instinctively knew when to push and when to pull and did both with love, honesty, encouragement and sensitivity.

Things do come to us through writing, and they are not always so intangible as insights. Moving our hands across the page, we make a handmade life. We tell the Universe what we like and what we don't like, what is bugging us and what is giving us delight. We tell the Universe and ourselves what we would like more of, what we would like less of, and through this clarity a shift occurs. Writing is a psychological as well as a physical activity. When I "clear my thoughts," I am literally rearranging my life itself.

Julia Cameron, *The Writer's Life*

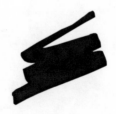

# A Gift the Self Can Give to the Soul

Healing is a complicated and dynamic process. Much has been written about the fact that complete healing means much more than physical improvement. Total healing must also encompass our spirit, our soul and our personal relationships. Unfortunately, the explosion of modern technology has caused modern health care professionals to emphasize the physical aspects of healing, which are concrete, easily understood and abundant. Yet, at the same time, most professionals struggle to help patients help themselves by finding additional tools that can heal a soul battered by emotional and physical illness.

Illness changes a patient's focus from routine life concerns to fears and doubts created by the experience of being ill. For someone accustomed to being healthy, feeling a loss of control, grieving over lost functions and opportunities, and the often disempowering and dehumanizing experience of being a patient is enormous.

It is well documented that stress negatively impacts healing. Recovery from cancer and serious infections such as AIDS and tuberculosis, and the management of diabetes, asthma and heart disease can be impeded by the effects of stress. How powerful, then, would be a tool that patients could use themselves to lower stress and promote healing.

*Write Your Self Well* is just such a tool. Journaling is a conscious process of examining the painful, confusing and joyous events in our lives. As a practicing internist, my experience with encouraging patients to use journaling as a means of self-expression and discovery has had, in many cases, a profound effect. Journaling has provided them solace, deepened their understanding of themselves and their illness, and created a catalyst for therapeutic discussion. In this way, a patient moves from being the subject of study for the therapeutic team to becoming an active team member. Healing then takes place, not just physically, but spiritually as well.

Relationships with family and friends often improve and even recovery times from physical insults such as surgery can decrease.

Ina Albert and Zoe Keithley have given us and those we care about a wonderful tool of empowerment and healing. It provides thoughtful, definitive guidance for those willing to explore the benefits of expressive writing. This is a gift the self can give to the soul.

Suzanne Daniell, M.D.
Whitefish, MT
December 14, 2003

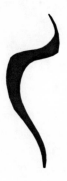

# "WHY JOURNAL?" YOU ASK

Millions of people store toxins of stress and trauma in their bodies that cause physical and emotional illness. This is no longer necessary. Medical research now proves that if you start writing, you'll start healing.

*Write Your Self Well…Journal Your Self to Health* is a guided tour inside you—a map that leads journalers into the past through inspiring quotes. The quotes on each page contain images designed to trigger memories by stimulating your senses.

The images may be happy or sad. They may remind you of great successes or bitter sadness. Or they may simply be pleasant memories. Whatever comes up is inviting you to go on a healing journey, knowing that the release of painful emotions and re-experiencing happiness and success has proven health benefits.

*Write Your Self Well* is uniquely designed to bring the benefits of expressive writing experienced by participants in twenty-plus years of clinical trials to all people suffering from chronic, acute or emotional illness.

# PART I

## Write Your Self Well . . .
### Journal Your Self to Health

"How do I know writing will help?
I don't even know what I'd write about."

*"Trust your memories—*

*the smell of brownies baking,*

*the sound of a train whistle.*

*Just see the images in your mind*

*and your hand will follow.*

# CHAPTER 1

# What Are the Health
# Benefits of Journaling?

Let's start our conversation with a scenario: You have been diagnosed with a painful chronic disease. Your mother ended her life badly crippled by the same illness after years of progressive pain. What can you do? Begin treatments. Follow doctor's orders. Keep your medical appointments. Try not to think about the future. Try not to think about the past. Stay close to family. Take it one day at a time. Pray.

Stop right there. Two of these commonplace nuggets of wisdom are truly bad choices for someone fighting illness. In fact, research has shown that one of them can actually impede your recovery.

The first bad piece of advice is: Try not to think about the future. We've all heard stories of unexplained and dramatic improvements in illness reported by people who tell of using their imaginations to creatively plan their futures. These stories of courageous people who refuse to despair demonstrate the very real linkage between the physical and mental/emotional worlds we call the mind-body connection that can powerfully influence the healing process.

The second bad piece of advice is: Don't think about the past; you're done with it. Most of us deal with only part of our life experience. We bury what we can't bear to look at—and with good reason. Then let's say we become sick and begin treatment. We have no idea that each of our mental/emotional burials has measurably decreased our chances for the recovery we desire.

Psychologists tell us that every unresolved issue begs, borrows or steals the energy we need for our own healing. We may feel it stored in stiff muscles, ulcers, depression, stress or back pain. And it is not only unhappy material that we bury. Often we have our reasons for denying ourselves access to happy experiences as well. When we don't confront these unresolved issues, we can't release the tremendous amounts of energy that are withheld from physical healing.

This would be a horrifying and daunting reality if it weren't for a powerful tool overlooked by most professionals and lay people, a tool able to break this deadlock. And you don't have to go to Amazon.com to order it because it's with you right here. The name healthcare professionals give to this wonder-working tool is "written disclosure." Some call it "expressive writing." Most of us call it "journaling."

Studies about the relationship of written disclosure to physical health have been underway for more than twenty years in the United States, Spain, Belgium, Japan, England, The Netherlands, Mexico and New Zealand. Through multiple clinical trials, medical science has shown that journaling promotes healing in strongly positive ways.

Writing as little as twenty minutes a day, every day, works. Writing about the past, present or future, about difficult problems in your life, about feelings, hopes, and dreams, will help you get better. Medical researchers don't know exactly how, but they know it will. That much has been proven.

"Okay. What makes you think I can write in a journal?" you ask.

The volunteers in written disclosure trials were not selected from a pool of seasoned journalers. We can assume that, like the rest of the population, some had no previous interest in journaling, and some actually had privately sworn never to be caught dead journaling. We can also assume a few had journaled before and liked it. Many people think of journaling as a woman's or an artist's thing, or something that records the progress of academics, sea captains or adventurers.

"That's not who I am," you say. "I don't do journaling. I can't even stand to write postcards, not even to my mother."

Okay. But you can talk. If you can talk, you can write. It's that easy. If you are a human being with a command of the alphabet, you can be good at journal writing.

Or you might say, "I'm fine with writing; I even like the idea—until I pick up a pen."

Ah yes, the fresh-page gag response, usually found as a subcategory of performance anxiety. We all know it well!

Remember, in your own journal you are performing for no one but yourself.

There's no way to do it wrong. There is no teacher to mark up your spelling or ask what happened to your semi-colons. No one will argue with your subject matter. There will be no snide remarks or probing questions. Your journal is private. You can go totally punctuation-free and fragment sentences silly. The more fun the better. It's your journal. The fact is that you must write the way you want about what you want for the process to work best.

In the next section we would like to share the basis of our journal process. But, perhaps you couldn't care less. You just want to go on to "How to Make Journaling Work Best for You." Feel free to skip ahead. You can always come back later.

# CHAPTER 2

## How Do We Know Journaling Works?

*"…the brightest spot of all is that at least I can write down all my thoughts and feelings; otherwise, I'd absolutely suffocate."*

Anne Frank, *The Diary of a Young Girl*

For over twenty years, medical researchers and psychologists have been studying the effects of written disclosure—journaling—on health. As a result, we know that expressing ourselves through writing has a measurably positive effect on both healthy people and patients suffering from illness, but we don't know why. What we do know is that expressive writing can shape, mold and recast human experience, and that rediscovering ourselves through writing about meaningful events in our lives can reduce stress and increase healing.

This is the internal work of the patient. Clinical trials have found that this work can have a positive and collaborative influence on the therapeutic work of the physician. *Write Your Self Well...Journal Your Self to Health* is based on solid research. Its purpose is to bring the results of clinical trials out of the lab and into the lives of those who would like to benefit from it. Here is some background you should know about:

In the mid-1980s, James W. Pennebaker, Ph.D., Professor of Psychology at the University of Texas at Austin, held a series of trials in which healthy individuals who wrote in journals about distressing experiences saw clear improvement in terms of fewer doctor visits. The study showed a strengthened immune system and a decrease in self-reported symptoms. His volunteer college students showed unexpected improvement in grades as well; and unemployed engineers found jobs before their non-disclosing out-of-work associates. In these trials, the physical and mental effects of journaling were surprising, pronounced and extensive.

Joshua M. Smyth, Ph.D., then at the University of North Dakota, conducted the first written disclosure experiment ever on people with chronic illness. Volunteers in 1998 were 112 patients with rheumatoid arthritis and asthma. His results appeared in *JAMA* (*Journal of the American Medical Association*) in 1999. Clear and dramatic health improvements in volunteers appeared after treatment. Smyth wrote that results were compelling. Not only were health effects reliably observed four months after the structured writing, but in addition, they appeared to be meaningful to the treatment process.

In Smyth's trial, the journaling process followed the research model of writing for twenty minutes on three consecutive days pioneered by Pennebaker. Some journalers wrote of common every day events; others wrote about deep and unresolved issues, often never before disclosed. Those who wrote about issues of deep personal concern or trauma achieved markedly higher results than those writing about surface events, although some of these also registered health benefits.

The same year, *The Writing Cure*, an anthology reporting research over the past two decades about written disclosure, strongly confirmed the effectiveness of expressive writing. Essays in the anthology also showed that any writing helps to some degree, that writing about happy topics produces good results as well as writing about trauma, though the latter produces the strongest outcomes.

Several studies showed that non-disclosure of trauma—suppressing distress—affects the body negatively. For example, a group of HIV-positive women who were also at risk for cervical cancer were found to have lower resistance to the disease than their counterparts who used disclosure as a coping mechanism. Even cities suffer. Another study showed that in cities where there have been natural disasters with no plan for post-disaster emotional processing, a marked increase in physical illness was reported in the next year.

USA Today broke the news of written disclosure experiments in an article entitled "You've got trauma, but writing can help" on July 1, 2002. This study demonstrated that writing e-mail to a confidential correspondent positively influenced 143 Texas A&M college students' well being.

*The Annals of Behavioral Medicine* (August 2002) published the findings of a University of Iowa study including 122 college students who wrote in their journals at least twice a week for four weeks about a painful experience. "Engagement of both thoughts and emotions while journaling about a stressful or traumatic experience can raise awareness of the benefits of the event," report Ullrich and Lutgendorf, the study's authors.

Expressive writing can release the suppressed pain and transform it into healing energy. While researchers and doctors continue to explore why journaling helps healing, positive physical results in ongoing research continue to be observed.

Participating in the creation of your own healing beyond what medical treatment and pharmaceuticals provide is the real possibility waiting for you.

# CHAPTER 3

## Journaling Can Work for You, Too

Let's start with some fundamental facts of life. All human beings form images in their minds and associate them with objects, responses or events in their lives. Through imaging—"seeing in the mind"—and associating, nature has created the ability for every human being think, speak and write.

Writer and educator John Schultz, creator of Story Workshop® approach, and behavioral psychologist Allan T. Paivio explain that our minds are fashioned by nature to image first, and it is the power of the image that coerces us into speech. 'Seeing in the mind' is a term created by John Schultz and includes memory, dreams, physical sensations and feelings. He explains that seeing in the mind tugs on language. Seeing in the mind and language working together help us find what we have to say.

Imaging is designed to be the natural bridge between thinking and speaking. Verbal processes are absent in imageless thought, Paivio says. Both Paivio and Schultz demonstrate that we use images to network associations and meanings in order to express and explain, to question and theorize, and come to understand our own and others' experiences of reality.

Images arise from a stimulus. Consider this example given by a journal writer. "Someone says 'Thanksgiving' and instantly I see my mother turn too fast from the oven and the turkey soar from the platter, then skid across the linoleum to bang into the dining room doors behind which sit dressed-up relatives with empty holiday plates. Next, I see her run the bottom of the bird under the faucet, pat it with a paper towel and plop it onto the platter. 'You can open the dining room doors,' she tells me."

Or you take in the smell of hot dust raised at your grandson's Little League game, and the second game of the 1963 World Series pops full-blown into your mind, complete with the baseball cap afloat above the cloud and tangle of arms and spiked feet at home plate. Then you're seeing a similar cloud and tangle of limbs, but it's the final game in your own high school regional tournament played on the hottest day of the year in 1947 in Muncie, Indiana.

The stimulus may be a sound, a sight, a smell, a movement or a touch. It may come from something that happens or something you read. You see "that other time" and all its details as if it were happening right now, and you may realize you had the same elated or difficult feelings then. That's imaging making its leaps and connections. The healing power of journaling lies in large part in these stimulus-evoked images and the way they trigger further memories and associations, calling the writer deeper into the scene. Paivio notes that the more concrete the memory, the greater its shelf life.

Words like "plastic spoon" and "gouge" unlock highly charged pictures and feelings, while abstract words like "wisdom" and "beauty" can't. Listening or reading, we can count on words that jump out at us or grab our attention to carry a load of meaning. A happy experience in adolescence, for instance, may never have been plumbed for its influence on us later in life. The fact that a strong image appeared, something we could see again clearly, tells us there is strong meaning for us. Some fragment of the memory lasted to be rediscovered through association tells us there is both strong meaning and intention in the memory to be recognized. The meaning in images compels us to connect with ourselves and with others in many ways.

These facts have practical value for someone using writing on the road to recovery. They guarantee that things that are important to us will appear for us to write about. And as we write, we continually release blocked energy that speeds our healing process.

Here's an example of a natural movement we make to find new energetic material. John Schultz calls it "the principle of whatever takes your attention." It is something you already use every day.

In a restaurant, you notice the man at the next table. Your eye is drawn to the way he holds his fork with the prongs facing down and how he piles mashed potatoes on the back, European style. This sight draws you sharply back to a Sunday dinner when you were seven and Uncle Helmut was visiting. Uncle Helmut's chair groaned under him, his plate groaned under his food. Uncle Helmut groaned as he ate. This image of Uncle Helmut raises a flash of old anger. At the end of the meal, there is one piece of pie left.

You ask for it, but you are only seven and insignificant. Uncle Helmut, who had three servings of everything and sweats profusely as he eats, gets the pie and you find you are still mad at your mother years later.

A single word in a book or conversation—pie or fork—may also take you to Uncle Helmet instantaneously. Then you may go on to other ways the family ignored you, or to a run-in with Uncle Helmut in your teens, or to the way you felt relieved in your twenties when they wheeled his casket into the church.

You never know what is going to take your attention, but you know it is significant or it wouldn't be able to work its way through the clutter continually impacting your consciousness to snag your mind. Notice the principle says, "what takes your attention," not "what you give your attention to." You are giving your attention to these words, but what is taking your attention might be that the sentences seem long, like toothpaste coming out of a tube. They go on and on—like the minister in church, or like your spouse as soon as you get in the door. You continue reading, but now you're thinking about how much of your life you are forced to spend listening to other people go on and on, especially people with supposed special stature, like your preacher or your boss.

Notice what took your attention was the feeling of being trapped in sentences going on and on, and that your imagination quickly supplied concrete images connected to the trapped and draggy feeling to make a bridge into other corresponding situations. If you had shunted aside the toothpaste image because it seemed silly or not relevant to you, you would have missed the pay dirt it was leading up to—realizing that you are sick and tired of putting up with some people's daily "on and ons."

Images appear in the wake of stimuli and are embedded with meaning. They are touchstones that lead us to further associations. They guarantee that things we care about will appear with no effort for us to write about. Things will come to us naturally because that's the way nature makes it work.

# CHAPTER 4

## How Can Journaling Work Best for Me?

*Write Your Self Well* is designed for where you are now.

You'll notice little writings on the pages above the journal pages. They are intended to stimulate images you can "see in your mind." You'll find these writings in different "voices" and in different forms, different people, situations, and walks of life. Flip through the journal pages. Whatever belongs to you will volunteer, intrude, or break in. It may not necessarily be something momentous—remember the toothpaste? But, it will have meaning.

When you feel that click that pulls on your feelings, or observe the vivid image erupting into your mind—trust it and start writing. Tell it any way you can. If, after a few minutes nothing more comes, begin flipping through the journal again until something else grabs you. Every image comes up on purpose—we know this—and it's not always to punch you in the nose. Maybe you don't see how what pulled you momentarily to a halt connects with anything. So what? You may not find out until you write. Anyway, your job is to write for twenty minutes a day, isn't it?

"What! You really meant twenty minutes? Every day? Are you crazy?"

Twenty minutes is what has worked in clinical trials. Listen, nobody said you had to make sense. Just write. Flip through and write. See what happens.

Every minute your pen moves, you are taking another step toward improving your health. Write as much as you can. Write a word, a list, a doodle, a stick figure. You are smarter than the average bear. We think you will find just flipping through will get you started; soon you will be using the little writings only occasionally.

Two other things are important for you to get the most from your journaling. The strongest results in clinical trials came for people who wrote about traumatic situations and found, through the writing, a way to resolve or integrate the trauma they experienced, or came to recognize some benefit from the experience. On every journaling page, we remind you to scan the page lightly and let something take your attention. Then, we ask what difference this has made in your life. Let yourself ask this or any other question that comes to mind. See what happens.

Notice the suggestions for different ways you can write. Writing in different forms is something like putting dough in the pastry gun and then forcing it through a unique cutout. Each time you write in a new form, you experience the content in a unique way. For instance, telling straight out about the accident you had on your bike when you were twelve will be one kind of story. It is quite another if told by your dog who happened to be there, or by your mangled bike.

Here are some suggestions for going about writing. See which of them appeals to you.

Styles/Techniques

A. <u>Draw. Draw and label</u>. Use stick figures if you're not Picasso. Tell the story; show the meaning, the feeling, the idea.

B. <u>Doodle</u> the meaning, the feeling, the memory.

C. <u>Tell whatever is happening straight out.</u>

D. <u>Use pen and ink images of your own</u> on the journal pages to prompt memories and feelings.

E. <u>Write a letter</u>. Tell about it in a letter to someone you trust. Or write to someone you have unfinished business or unstated issues with. Write to someone you want to acknowledge or to thank. Write to someone you want to question.

F. <u>Dialogue</u>. In Progoff's Intensive Journaling Workshop, dialogue is suggested for opening up new or old material. Dialogue with someone or something—your job, your pet, the government, ambition, fear, resentment, religion, a new idea, your past, or your future. You are one half of the dialogue; the other half is Work, or Future, or Fear of Failure. Let your self-chosen dialogue partner speak. You may be surprised that Religion and Ambition each have a distinct voice and are more than ready to go at it with you.

G. <u>Hold onto the image or scene</u>. If you keep attending to it, you'll notice the image changing. It will begin to unfold itself and give you more information. Keep watching it develop, and write whatever you notice or whatever comes to you.

H. Make lists. List objects, sounds, smells, sensations, names of people, places, games, tools, dance steps, holidays, the birthdays in the family, phone numbers. List the things that give you pleasure—go through the alphabet; or list the things you resent—go through the alphabet. That should use up a few twenty-minute sessions.

I. Circle list items. Using the Principle of Whatever Takes Your Attention, go over a list you've made. Circle any item on the list that pops out at you. There may be several. Write whatever you have to say about each one.

J. Random write. Educational innovator Anne Schultz recommends that you just start writing. It is unusual to write, even nonsensically, for as much as ten minutes without something of genuine interest coming to your attention. Reread your writing of previous days. Circle anything that pops out at you. Write more about that.

K. Write a poem. You don't have to be a poet. Write whatever your idea of a poem is. No one's going to see it anyway.

L. Write a song lyric. Take a tune you know well with a familiar lyric—"Frère Jacques," "America the Beautiful," "Itsy Bitsy Teeny Weenie Yellow Polka-dot

Bikini," "Take Me Out to the Ball Game," "This Land Is Your Land," "Yesterday"—and write a new lyric telling a story, your feelings around a subject, speaking to someone you love or don't.

M. <u>Write in your own voice</u>. Say things whatever way is comfortable and appropriate for your subject and your feelings. The language you like is the perfect language to use. And nobody is going to read what you wrote unless you choose to let them.

N. <u>Flip through the springboard writings for memory and feeling associations</u>. Notice whatever tugs on you. The same written image or drawing can produce different responses in you on different days. Trust the tug. It doesn't happen by accident.

O. <u>Others</u>? Create your own style.

More often than not, one writing leads to another. Of course, this is the best situation because when you hit a groove or discover a rich vein of ore, you get up a head of steam. Then you can follow it as long as it is producing for you. Later, you can go back to using the flip-through method and the model writings when you've exhausted all the connections.

When you fill your journal, you will find you have created a 3-D picture of the place you are in your life right now. It may be the beginning of a set as you start the next journal. Start where you are. Write a little. Write a lot. Write twenty minutes every day. Write.

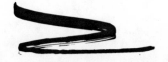

# CHAPTER 5

## Quotes and Images

*"In a few hours after being admitted to the hospital,
Rusanov had lost his whole status in life, his honors,
and his plans for the future, and had become 168
pounds of warm white flesh that did not know what
would happen to it tomorrow."*

Alexander Solzhenitsyn, *The Cancer Ward*

In *The Cancer Ward,* Rusanov's sudden loss of identity not only
made him invisible to the hospital staff, but to himself as well.
Reduced to an object—worse—an ailing, defective object. He
is alone. Weak. Naked.

Think of the images this passage suggests. A revealing hospital gown, lying on a gurney in a hospital hallway. Being renamed an Arthritis—Asthma—you name the disease—patient. Cold sheets, narrow beds, smells of disinfectants.

The quotes that follow have many voices and reflect different life experiences, writing styles and means of expression. All of them are written to trigger sensations and personal memories to help journalers "see in the mind".

1. <u>Feelings about treatment</u> pain and anger need to be expressed. Writing about medical treatment allows emotions to vent:

   *"They were drawing this big tube out of me and it hurt so much I started to cry. The nurse didn't like that. I could see she was afraid it might bother the doctor, and she told me to pull myself together. If I'd had the strength I would have told her I was pulling myself together by crying instead of fainting."*

2. <u>Letters</u> can evoke similar frustrating experiences:

*Dear Mr. Crabbetree,*

*You still owe me $150 cleaning deposit from June, 1974, in Monterey. You knew the sundeck furniture had rotted through before we ever moved in. We kept your cheap place spotless, and it wasn't my wife's fault the color came off the counter when she scoured it. But, I learned a lesson from you, buddy. Make a list, just like with the rental car people. That way I won't get taken for a ride again. Zorro*

3. <u>Dreams</u> like a childhood nightmare are a frequent source of frightening images filled with fear and guilt. Yet they are rich with metaphors that beg to be explored:

*"I dreamed my sister pulled up her shirt to show me her back. She was crying. There were horrible big pimples on her back. She asked me to squeeze them. When I did, horrible big black spiders came crawling out."*

4. <u>Painful memories</u> may touch internally held issues of fear and shame and bring them to the surface for exploration and healing:

*"I remember my father came drunk to my high school graduation. My friends gave me these funny looks. Nobody knew what to say. He was always showing up drunk at the wrong time. I couldn't wait to get out of that house."*

5. <u>Poems</u> can encapsulate feelings and experiences and can be fun:

# Sex

So tired of saying yes to him.

No matter how I'm feeling.

You'd think he'd see my attitude.

And he'd hit the ceiling.


But no. He's used to the routine.

It never seems to bore him.

He's comfortable the way it is,

So I turn on my side and ignore him.

6. <u>Recipes</u> can give the perspective of humor and offer a place of discovery:

# Recipe for Heartburn

Take one argument and tear it into twenty

small pieces. Spice each piece with a mean memory

and stick it on a skewer. Cook over a hot temper

for fifteen minutes on each side. Serve this

same meal every day for a month.

7. <u>Song lyrics</u> offer a creative and non-threatening way of dealing with serious issues that stimulate rhythmic and auditory senses:

How I wish I could be younger

Get things done, have some fun.

But, instead of that I'm useless

Old and grey and toothless

And can't chew gum, can't chew gum.

(To the tune of Frére Jacques)

8. <u>Dialogue</u>, talking with your intimate self, with your mirror or with others sharpens our sense of internal speaking and listening:

*"You know, Dad, when I'm doing work around the house, I think about when you died. Seventies is not that old now. I've still got lots of time. I'll fight this thing and I'll win."*

*"You've got to do something! Your mother keeps getting out of bed in the middle of the night. I found her at two in the morning sitting in the stairwell on the twenty-fifth floor of our apartment house. She could have killed herself. I'm at my wits' end. You're her daughter. You've got to do something!"*

9. <u>One-liners</u>. High impact statements such as these are powerful. They reflect a deep honesty and truth:

*"The doctor told me that I have six months to live."*

*"I just don't love you anymore. I want a divorce."*

# PART II

## Write Your Self Well...
### Journal Your Self to Health

"Tell everyone you need time to yourself.

Find a good pen or pencil.

Find a quiet, comfortable place.

Close your eyes, take a deep breath and relax.

This time belongs to you alone.

Now write."

# CHAPTER 6

## Suggestions for Journaling

The quotes on each page contain images designed to trigger memories by stimulating your senses. They may be happy or sad. They may remind you of great successes or bitter grief. Or they may simply be pleasant memories. Whatever comes up is inviting you to go on a healing journey, knowing that the release of painful emotions and re-experiencing happiness and success has proven health benefits.

If you follow these suggestions carefully, you'll get the best results:

• Just flip through the pages of quotes as John Schultz suggests.

- Let your eyes scan the page lightly.

- When you feel that personal *click*; when something 'pops out' or 'tugs' on your feelings, or you see a vivid image erupting into your mind—trust it and start writing immediately about whatever it reminds you of in the space below the quotes.

- Tell how you feel about it any way you can.

- Then ask yourself what difference it has made in your life.

- If, after a few minutes, nothing more comes, begin flipping through the pages again until something else grabs you.

- Every image that comes up in your mind comes up on purpose. Maybe you don't see how what pulled you momentarily to a halt connects with anything. So what? You may not find out until you start to write.

- Let yourself be creative. You can draw, doodle or write song lyrics to express the image you see in your mind. Write a letter, a dialogue, make a list, or any other means of expression that you can think of.

- Just stick with your image when it comes. See it in your mind. Let it take you and go with it!

- No matter what comes up—happy or sad—let it happen. Feeling emotional release is a good thing and will help you get healthier!

- Use your Personal Healing Chart to Graph your progress.

- Now have at it!

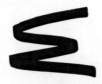

# CHAPTER 7

## Write Your Self Well Journal

Guidepost: Scan the page lightly. When something "pops out" or "tugs" on you, start writing about whatever it reminds you of immediately. Then ask yourself what difference it has made in your life.

"That day at grandma and grandpa's house,

when I shouted something I thought was funny,

I learned it wasn't safe to be myself in front of grown-ups."

"When Dad tried to teach me to drive a stick shift,

I bucked the car all the way down the street.

The next day he asked someone else to teach me on

their car."

"I'm going to put an electric fence around my bed. Then they won't be able to get near me with their needles and probes, their stethoscopes and blood pressure cuffs, their portable X-rays and EKG machines. When I get home, I'll take the fence down and let people in."

_____

_____

_____

_____

_____

_____

_____

_____

_____

_____

_____

_____

_____

_____

_____

_____

_____

_____

_____

_____

_____

_____

_____

_____

_____

_____

_____

_____

_____

_____

_____

_____

_____

_____

_____

_____

_____

_____

_____

_____

_____

Scan the page lightly. When something "pops out" or "tugs" on you, start writing immediately about whatever it reminds you of. Then ask yourself what difference it has made in your life.

"Farfel was all black and white fluff when I first held her in

my hands. She was the first puppy I ever held—

warm and squirmy, smelling like a fur ball."

"I remember my father came drunk to my high school

graduation. He was always showing up drunk at the wrong

time."

"The first time our gang went to a bar,

I put on lots of makeup so people would think I was older.

But, they still asked for ID, and I never did

get a drink that night."

_____

_____

_____

_____

_____

_____

_____

_____

_____

_____

_____

_____

_____

_____

_____

_____

_____

_____

_____

_____

_____

_____

_____

_____

_____

_____

Scan the page lightly. When something "pops out" or "tugs" on you, start writing immediately about whatever it reminds you of. Then ask yourself what difference it has made in your life.

Big ring,

Shining ring,

With a heart of stone.

Where did you go?

Back to the store where he bought you,

Or on some other moon-eyed gal's finger.

"So, Truth, where are you hiding?

If it is a truth that I am old, why do I still feel so young? If it is a truth that death is a natural part of life, why am I so frightened of dying? If it is a truth that our memory will live on in our good deeds, why can't my children remember to call once a week?

Truth, where are you hiding?"

_____

_____

_____

_____

_____

_____

_____

_____

_____

_____

_____

_____

_____

_____

_____

_____

_____

_____

_____

_____

_____

_____

_____

_____

_____

Scan the page lightly. When something "pops out" or "tugs" on you, start writing immediately about whatever it reminds you of. Then ask yourself what difference it has made in your life.

# Soul Foods

Fry Bread               Gefilte Fish            Lefse

Gnocchi                 Grits                   Matzo

Peanut Butter and Jelly Humus                  Chorizos

Mole                    Chocolate Chips         Frijoles y arroz

Enchiladas              Roasted Marshmallows Cat Fish

_____

_____

_____

_____

_____

_____

_____

_____

_____

_____

_____

Scan the page lightly. When something "pops out" or "tugs" on you, start writing immediately about whatever it reminds you of. Then ask yourself what difference it has made in your life.

"I can still smell the dune grass, dry and sticky like tack.

The sand between my toes."

"It seems like I will never get well.

One problem just leads to another and I feel like all my systems

are breaking down—like a motor that is rusting away."

"When I opened the front door of the new house

and stepped outside, the whole world smelled like

a Christmas tree."

"In this dream, my wife would be telling me I should lose

weight. But there I'd be as thin as a rail. In the dream I'd think,

'Can't you see I'm skinny?'

But she'd go on and on, yet she'd be fat as a house."

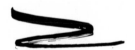

Scan the page lightly. When something "pops out" or "tugs" on you, start writing immediately about whatever it reminds you of. Then ask yourself what difference it has made in your life.

"An old skate key in the back of a drawer.

I can almost feel the

bumpy cement under my skate wheels."

"We played Spin-the-Bottle. When the bottle pointed to me,

Jimmy took me in the closet and kissed me.

It was wet and icky."

"Leaning back, I let the speedboat pull me up.
Skimming across the water back and forth over the wake,
my arms stretched out in front of me. I was flying. Flying!"

"Oh, God! It's so dark in my room and I don't have
enough air. I can't catch my breath. And my chest is closing
up. I'm all wet. Hot. Cold. Mommy! It's happening again!
Mommy!!!!!!"

_____

_____

_____

_____

_____

_____

_____

_____

_____

_____

_____

_____

_____

_____

_____

_____

_____

_____

_____

_____

_____

_____

_____

_____

_____

_____

Scan the page lightly. When something "pops out" or "tugs" on you, start writing immediately about whatever it reminds you of. Then ask yourself what difference it has made in your life.

# Memories

| | | |
|---|---|---|
| Nancy Drew | Pooh Bear | The Prince |
| Wendy | Good Night Moon | Bambi |
| Capt. Marvel | Kermit | Narnia Chronicles |
| Elmer Fudd | Roadrunner | Wonder Woman |

_____

_____

_____

_____

_____

_____

_____

_____

_____

_____

_____

_____

_____

Scan the page lightly. When something "pops out" or "tugs" on you, start writing immediately about whatever it reminds you of. Then ask yourself what difference it has made in your life.

"When my dad died he was in his seventies.

I've still got plenty of time. I'm not ready yet.

But when I am, God, take me fast."

       "It was like Woodstock.

       All the hippies with tie-dyed shirts and long

       scraggly hair, smoking dope, laying in the sun and

       touching each other while the music played so loud

       my whole body vibrated."

"I've gotten so into the doc and the gal who brings meds, or the one who changes IVs and the Asian trick who brings my tray. I know what to say to them, how to joke. But when my daughter comes, I haven't got a single thing to say to her because she doesn't live in this place. And I feel embarrassed and guilty, like I gave her place in the family away."

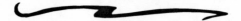

_____

_____

_____

_____

_____

_____

_____

_____

_____

_____

_____

_____

_____

_____

_____

_____

_____

_____

_____

_____

_____

_____

_____

_____

Scan the page lightly. When something "pops out" or "tugs" on you, start writing immediately about whatever it reminds you of. Then ask yourself what difference it has made in your life.

"I'm glad I got the bed near the window.

I can feel the warm sun on my hands and see the sky."

"Sundays we would visit Grandma.

We'd sit in her musty smelling parlor on the cut velvet love

seat and drink her special lemonade with

real crushed strawberries in it."

"terrible terrible terrible terrible terrible terrible

terrible terrible food

tedious tedious tedious tedious tedious tedious tedious tedious

tedious pain

hot hot hot hot hot hot urine

furry furry furry furry furry furry furry mouth

cold cold cold cold cold cold bedpan

long long long long long long long long long days

whacky whacky whacky whacky whacky sleep

private private private private private private private—not!"

"DON'T TOUCH ME!"

_____

_____

_____

_____

_____

_____

_____

_____

_____

_____

_____

_____

_____

_____

_____

_____

_____

_____

_____

_____

_____

_____

Scan the page lightly. When something "pops out" or "tugs" on you, start writing immediately about whatever it reminds you of. Then ask yourself what difference it has made in your life.

"My mom was just sitting up in bed, waiting for breakfast...

Then she coughed and fell over. That's how she died."

"I remember my knobby wool shirt,

how it felt in my fingers and on my face when I rubbed it—

safe and warm and familiar.

I could sure use that shirt right now."

"When I drink green tea, I think of Grandma

and remember how she let it steep in the pot.

Then she put a silver strainer on top of her

cup to catch the tea leaves.

In those days, she was the only person I knew

who drank green tea."

_____

_____

_____

_____

_____

_____

_____

_____

_____

_____

_____

_____

_____

_____

_____

_____

_____

_____

_____

_____

_____

_____

_____

_____

_____

_____

_____

Scan the page lightly. When something "pops out" or "tugs" on you, start writing immediately about whatever it reminds you of. Then ask yourself what difference it has made in your life.

# Old Memories

| | | |
|---|---|---|
| Iron skillet | Cod liver oil | Ration stamps |
| Oil cloth | Lisle stockings | Hit Parade |
| Party lines | Storm sashes | Mustard plasters |
| Milkman | Bobbie pins | American Bandstand |

_____

_____

_____

_____

_____

_____

_____

_____

_____

_____

_____

_____

_____
_____
_____
_____
_____
_____
_____
_____
_____
_____
_____
_____
_____
_____
_____
_____
_____
_____
_____
_____
_____

Scan the page lightly. When something "pops out" or "tugs" on you, start writing immediately about whatever it reminds you of. Then ask yourself what difference it has made in your life.

Recipe for Heartburn

Tear one argument into twenty small pieces.

Spice each piece with mean memory and stick on a skewer.

Cook over hot temper for fifteen minutes to a side.

Serve this same meal every day of your life.

"I see the ocean and the waves for the first time and think,

'It really is white with foam!'

And the white silky sand squeaks as my feet skim over it.

And the fishy, salty, seaweed smell of it all catches my breath.

And my feet sink into the wet sand at the water's edge.

And I push into the waves.

They take me and we play together."

_____

_____

_____

_____

_____

Scan the page lightly. When something "pops out" or "tugs" on you, start writing immediately about whatever it reminds you of. Then ask yourself what difference it has made in your life.

"When they told me he died, I shut everyone out and started

rocking back and forth. I just couldn't stop rocking, waiting

for the tears to start."

"I still love Elvis.

I keep his picture up in my room

and save all the records and movie magazines

from when he was alive.

My accountant is an Elvis freak, too.

He has a full-size costumed Elvis in his office

and signed photographs everywhere."

"Every Saturday afternoon, my cousin Jocelyn

and I would get out our movie magazines.

We'd cut out the pictures of the stars

and paste them into our scrapbook.

Then I'd pretend I was Katharine Hepburn

and she would be Elizabeth Taylor."

Scan the page lightly. When something "pops out" or "tugs" on you, start writing immediately about whatever it reminds you of. Then ask yourself what difference it has made in your life.

"I wish I could wake up and this would all be over."

"Every once in while, I feel a light tug on my fishing line, but wait until it gets stronger. Then I set the lure and this big, beautiful bass jumps a foot out of the water and the sun makes a rainbow on him before he plunges back again and starts swimming for it. He keeps me out there for almost an hour, playing me the way I play him."

"This is how you make a burrito.
You put hamburger, beans, cheese and salsa in the middle of the tortilla. Then fold it in a half moon and tuck in the ends so nothing leaks out. Then roll the long, closed side toward the curved edges, but first you tuck the top layer of the tortilla under the filling a little.
Then roll it until the curved edges are on the bottom.
Most people don't know how to do that."

_____

_____

_____

_____

_____

_____

_____

_____

_____

_____

_____

_____

_____

_____

_____

_____

_____

_____

_____

_____

_____

_____

Scan the page lightly. When something "pops out" or "tugs" on you, start writing immediately about whatever it reminds you of. Then ask yourself what difference it has made in your life.

"When I let my hair go gray, I felt free.

All those years of dyed hair—for what?"

"When I was sixteen, I decided to light up like Mom and Dad.

Then Mom smelled the smoke and pushed

open the door to my room.

She had such a sad look on her face."

"My Dad's golfing buddy came to dinner a lot.

He'd always come up to my room to tuck me in.

He'd touch me in places where he shouldn't

have and I was scared to tell."

_____

_____

_____

_____

_____

_____

Scan the page lightly. When something "pops out" or "tugs" on you, start writing immediately about whatever it reminds you of. Then ask yourself what difference it has made in your life.

# Heroes and Villains

| | | |
|---|---|---|
| Harry Truman | Saddam Hussein | Eleanor Roosevelt |
| Fidel Castro | Joe McCarthy | Benito Juarez |
| Ariel Sharon | Hillary Clinton | George W. Bush |
| Martin Luther King, Jr. | Neil Armstrong | Nelson Mandela |
| Sandra Day O'Connor | JFK | Princess Di |

_____

_____

_____

_____

_____

_____

_____

_____

_____

_____

_____

_____

_____

_____

_____

_____

_____

_____

_____

_____

_____

Scan the page lightly. When something "pops out" or "tugs" on you, start writing immediately about whatever it reminds you of. Then ask yourself what difference it has made in your life.

"How do you plead?" asked the judge.

"I gave her a twenty, but she gave me back change for a ten. I told her I gave her a twenty. She said no. Then she said she'd have to count her cash drawer. She put my groceries behind the counter and took me with the cash drawer to the manager's office figuring I lied because I was old and had buttons off my coat. In the end, the manager never said a word, just handed me the other ten. I said I wanted my groceries. He said, 'Oh yeah, give her those.'"

_____

_____

_____

_____

_____

_____

_____

_____

Scan the page lightly. When something "pops out" or "tugs" on you, start writing immediately about whatever it reminds you of. Then ask yourself what difference it has made in your life.

"Why do I worry so much about being late for my doctor's appointment? I always have to wait for him. Isn't my time worth anything? Maybe I should charge him my hourly rate."

"It was rush hour on the Thruway. I looked down to check the address of this new place I was driving to. When I looked up, I was right on top of the car ahead of me. I jammed on my brakes, but I hit him anyway. My car had its face hanging off, but he only had a broken taillight."

"I came back from lunch and Tim said, 'Mr. Burnell wants to see you.' I was glad I came back from lunch on time. His secretary showed me right in. He hardly looked up. 'We won't be needing you anymore,' he said. 'This will be your last day.'
It was like someone sucked all the air out of my body.
All I could think was to get out of there.
I didn't want to get sick in front of him."

Scan the page lightly. When something "pops out" or "tugs" on you, start writing immediately about whatever it reminds you of. Then ask yourself what difference it has made in your life.

"I got a job busing tables—me and all these young kids. I

needed the money. I was drop dead

tired at first, but pretty soon I was better

than all of them."

"She grabbed me and put me in the closet.

She said that was where you put bad boys.

I begged, 'Please don't put me in there.'

But she closed the door and I was scared that

skeletons or snakes might reach out and grab me,

so I kicked and kicked the door and yelled,

'Let me out!'"

"Living way out here so far away from family,

I feel disconnected and lonely."

_____

_____

_____

_____

_____

_____

_____

_____

_____

_____

_____

_____

_____

_____

_____

_____

_____

_____

_____

_____

_____

_____

_____

_____

_____

Scan the page lightly. When something "pops out" or "tugs" on you, start writing immediately about whatever it reminds you of. Then ask yourself what difference it has made in your life.

"I don't understand what they're saying in their alphabet soup medical language, but I feel safer here than at home. Just wish they would explain things to me."

"My parents made me go on this stupid canoe trip last summer. Like a camp way out in the sticks. All we did was carry all this stuff through the woods and swat mosquitoes. Nothing to drink but Kool-Aid. We had to put our own tents up and were awake half the night. Every time someone turned over, the stupid tent fell down."

"He was like a big bear coming at me,
his beer gut hanging out and his eyes bloodshot.
'You always got an answer for your old man,' he'd yell.
I'd dodge, but he'd knock me up against the wall and then it'd
be like red-hot shovels smashing my ears and jaw and nose.
I'd feel the blood spurt.
But I wouldn't give him the satisfaction of an
answer. I wouldn't cry either or hit him back.
I didn't hit my father."

Scan the page lightly. When something "pops out" or "tugs" on you, start writing immediately about whatever it reminds you of. Then ask yourself what difference it has made in your life.

"I really need to feel a human hand touch me without an IV

needle or syringe in it.

I need to have my hair stroked the way Mom used to."

"I stuck my thumb out and held it high in the air on the side of the highway to hitch a ride. My friend was scared and stood behind me. An older couple stopped to pick us up. As soon as we got into the car they started lecturing us about how dangerous it was to hitch hike, and did our parents know where we were, and on and on."

"The movie made me so sad that I couldn't wait

to get home and pull my puppy up on my bed,

and feel her lick my face and stroke her fur."

_____

_____

_____

_____

_____

_____

_____

_____

_____

_____

_____

_____

_____

_____

_____

_____

_____

_____

_____

_____

_____

_____

_____

_____

_____

Scan the page lightly. When something "pops out" or "tugs" on you, start writing immediately about whatever it reminds you of. Then ask yourself what difference it has made in your life.

"Imagine you are picking up one end of a big sturdy rope. Take a minute to let someone else appear holding the other end. Notice a big sloppy mud hole between you, the rope passing over it. Begin pulling on your end of the rope. Really put muscle into it. Feel the strong resistance on the other end. Who is the other person? What is this struggle about? What is the mud hole? Hang in and keep pulling."

*"I smell bread baking."*

"Here he comes. I know the doctor's footsteps. Oops. They've stopped. He must be talking to the nurse before he comes to see me.

That's it! He's checking my chart.

I hear him coming…. clop, clop, clop.

It's getting louder. Clop, clop, clop, clop.

He's not stopping. He's going right past my door.

Clop, clop, clop, cloppppppp."

Scan the page lightly. When something "pops out" or "tugs" on you, start writing immediately about whatever it reminds you of. Then ask yourself what difference it has made in your life.

# Movie Stars

| | | |
|---|---|---|
| John Lennon | Bruce Willis | Marx Brothers |
| Tom Hanks | Bette Davis | Britney Spears |
| George Clooney | Jorge Negreti | Judy Garland |
| Jack Lemmon | John Wayne | Sean Connery |
| Hugh Grant | Meryl Streep | Clint Eastwood |

_____

_____

_____

_____

_____

_____

_____

_____

_____

_____

_____

_____

_____

_____

Scan the page lightly. When something "pops out" or "tugs" on you, start writing immediately about whatever it reminds you of. Then ask yourself what difference it has made in your life.

"My friend had gone on a diet, writing down everything he ate each day. 'I even have to write down the Wheat Thins, how many servings,' he told me. 'Before, I used to think a box was one serving.' I tried not to let my eyes get big or laugh."

"When our cat Max was dying, just before we took him to be put to sleep, he came staggering up to each member of our family, one by one, and said good-bye. My husband put a pillow on the floor and Max curled up on it. He placed the tip of his tail over his nose and never moved from that position again."

"She's so beautiful that I can't take my eyes off her. She feels me staring at her, looks me straight in the eye and turns away."

_____

_____

_____

_____

Scan the page lightly. When something "pops out" or "tugs" on you, start writing immediately about whatever it reminds you of. Then ask yourself what difference it has made in your life.

"I was on the Indiana in WW II—the radioman. My station was directly under this big pipe that carried live steam. Every time we would be receiving enemy fire, I couldn't help picturing the pipe exploding with me beneath it, and
live steam scalding me to death."


"I used to get lost a lot. I didn't want to ask anyone for directions. One time I must have walked for hours. All the buildings kept looking familiar. Finally, I broke
down and called my dad at work. He told me to go read the street signs, and when I told him what they said he got very quiet. Then he said, 'Don't move. And don't talk to
anyone. I'll be there in twenty minutes.'"

_____

_____

_____

_____

_____

Scan the page lightly. When something "pops out" or "tugs" on you, start writing immediately about whatever it reminds you of. Then ask yourself what difference it has made in your life.

"I have this job at an ice cream parlor in San Diego. They've got me on a ladder scrubbing the outside of the building, when this guy comes along and stops and looks up. We recognize each other from law school. We graduated together. 'Oh great,' he says, 'we're supposed to be making sixty grand a year and you're scrubbing restaurant walls and I'm living in my car.'"

"We're walking down a street in Paris to meet our parents and my brother keeps rubbing his hand along my leg as we walk. I keep moving away, but he keeps on doing it. Finally, I say, 'Stop that, Tim.' He looks at me all innocence, like I'm crazy. 'Stop what?' he asks. A few steps later he does it again. I'm getting desperate, so I say, like a first grader, 'OK, I'm telling Mom and Dad.' That stops him.

_____

_____

_____

_____

_____
_____
_____
_____
_____
_____
_____
_____
_____
_____
_____
_____
_____
_____
_____
_____
_____
_____
_____
_____
_____

Scan the page lightly. When something "pops out" or "tugs" on you, start writing immediately about whatever it reminds you of. Then ask what difference it has made in your life.

# Memories

| | | |
|---|---|---|
| Elvis | Frank Sinatra | The Beatles |
| Count Basie | Michael Jackson | Julio Iglesias |
| Billie Holiday | Madonna | Tina Turner |
| Duke Ellington | Leonard Bernstein | Rodgers and Hart |
| Crosby, Stills and Nash | Barbra Streisand | Luis Miguel |
| Lena Horne | Benny Goodman | Rolling Stones |

_____

_____

_____

_____

_____

_____

_____

_____

_____

_____

_____

_____

Scan the page lightly. When something "pops out" or "tugs" on you, start writing immediately about whatever it reminds you of. Then ask yourself what difference it has made in your life.


Dear Aunt Kate,

Home from the beach, Uncle Joe at the back door asking to see the bottoms of our feet. They'd be covered with black tar. He'd rub it off with kerosene and we'd hold our noses. Remember?

Love, Mary


"She didn't have to be so snotty about it. After all, it was her idea to have the party in the first place. Then she had to do everything herself, making it look like there wasn't a living human being who could set a table as well as she could or lay out a few cheese and crackers so they looked decent. Everything I suggested was wrong. After she said, 'That will never work,' or 'Are you color blind?' for the twelfth time, I figured I'd let her do it all herself."

_____

_____

_____

_____

Scan the page lightly. When something "pops out" or "tugs" on you, start writing immediately about whatever it reminds you of. Then ask yourself what difference it has made in your life.

"I transferred to a new high school in tenth grade.

One day between classes, these kids came and stood

around me in a circle and asked me why I wasn't going to the

football games. Didn't I like the school? Didn't I have school spirit? I

didn't like the school, but I wasn't stupid enough to say so.

Like a jerk, I showed up at the next game

and was disgusted with myself for knuckling under."

"Ever since the fire, the smell of smoke starts my heart pounding.

I hear that crackle again and my daughter screaming,

Daddy, Daddy!!!"

"They told me when I got home she'd been run down by a guy

having a stroke. She was pushed right through the windshield.

I put my hands over my ears, trying not to hear

what it must have felt like."

_____

_____

_____

_____

_____

Scan the page lightly. When something "pops out" or "tugs" on you, start writing immediately about whatever it reminds you of. Then ask yourself what difference it has made in your life.

"Get away from me and leave me alone!

You really don't care about me."

"I was three or four, Mom's apple pie was cooling, but there were flies coming on it, so I shooed them off and the pie fell on the floor. Mom picked it up and smacked it on my head. She yelled, 'You might as well have all of it,' and left me standing there."

"Having a baby was scary. I was afraid of the pain,

but I wanted to be brave.

They tell you that you forget the pain afterwards and only

remember holding the baby in your arms.

But I still remember the pain."

_____

_____

_____

_____

_____

_____

_____

Scan the page lightly. When something "pops out" or "tugs" on you, start writing immediately about whatever it reminds you of. Then ask yourself what difference it has made in your life.

"When my neighbor won the lottery, I wondered why he should have all the luck. It made me remember the raffle in grammar school when I wanted to win the model airplane and did odd jobs to get money for tickets, and then a girl won it."

"I went to the store to buy clothes for my first grandchild—
the first girl!
I stood looking at all those dresses
and burst into tears."

"My Cary died in an accident hit by a drunk driver.
I try not to think what that felt like."

_____

_____

_____

_____

_____

_____

Scan the page lightly. When something "pops out" or "tugs" on you, start writing immediately about whatever it reminds you of. Then ask yourself what difference it has made in your life.

Dear Mom and Dad,

I still remember tearing the wrapping paper away, ripping off the lid, beating back the tissue, smelling the smooth white leather and seeing the shiny blades of those ice skates. I wanted to leave all the rest of the gifts unopened and head straight for the skating pond.

Love, Joan

"The smell of a fresh ripe peach on a hot summer day. Biting through the fuzzy skin and feeling the sugar sweet juice dribble down my chin."

"I was a poor kid growing up, so getting that first job in an office and wearing a shirt and tie made me feel like a million bucks."

_____

_____

_____

_____

Scan the page lightly. When something "pops out" or "tugs" on you, start writing immediately about whatever it reminds you of. Then ask yourself what difference it has made in your life.

# Sports Heroes

Peggy Fleming

Billie Jean King

Picabo Street

Michael Jordan

Man O' War

Pele

Vince Lombardi

Arnold Palmer

Johnny Unitas

Gordy Howe

Jon Claude Keely

Muhammad Ali

Bruce Jenner

Mickey Mantle

Dorothy Hamil

_____

_____

_____

_____

_____

_____

_____

_____

_____

_____

_____

_____

_____

_____

Scan the page lightly. When something "pops out" or "tugs" on you, start writing immediately about whatever it reminds you of. Then ask yourself what difference it has made in your life.

"I remember those teenage Saturday afternoons going downtown and standing in front of a department store until we saw a middle-aged woman—usually with her mind full of shopping. We'd drop back some steps behind and follow her until we sensed her deciding to confront us. Then we'd split and find another victim."

"I escaped from Cuba over forty-five years ago
with five dollars in my pocket.
Now I have a good marriage, a nice home, a successful business
and healthy grandchildren. I guess I did all right."

_____

_____

_____

_____

_____

_____

_____

_____

_____

_____

_____

_____

_____

_____

_____

_____

_____

_____

_____

_____

_____

_____

_____

_____

_____

_____

_____

_____

_____

Scan the page lightly. When something "pops out" or "tugs" on you, start writing immediately about whatever it reminds you of. Then ask yourself what difference it has made in your life.

"Ding. Dingdingding … Ding Ding … Dingdingding … Ding Ding … Dingdingding …Ding ... Doctor Westover. Doctor Westover. Ding …Dingdingding …Ding … Ding … Dingdingding … Ding …Doctor Westover … All day."

"My new baby felt so warm and soft cradled in my arms, like fine silk still warm from being ironed. It puckered its lips looking for something to suck on and I could see its pink tongue waiting to taste the nipple."

"Nobody tells you about a hard-on until it's happening. You're in school or at church and what's this? Up goes the oar! My old man never told me a thing, and not a thing in school. The guys I snuck smokes with told me or I might still think I was a medical case."

_____

_____

_____

_____

_____

_____

_____

_____

_____

_____

_____

_____

_____

_____

_____

_____

_____

_____

_____

_____

_____

_____

_____

_____

_____

_____

_____

_____

_____

_____

_____

Scan the page lightly. When something "pops out" or "tugs" on you, start writing immediately about whatever it reminds you of. Then ask yourself what difference it has made your life.

"A-Tisket, A-Tasket, My Little Yellow Basket.

I played that song on my Victrola a thousand times to hear

Ella Fitzgerald's voice and pretended

my Raggedy Ann was singing."


"Mother saved pennies in a box in the bottom drawer of her

dresser for the missions. One day I decided there were so

many pennies she would never miss a few handfuls, but she

did, and she blamed my brother for taking them. He was so

hurt that he went into the yard and tore the three dollars he

had gotten for allowance to bits. From the window upstairs, I

watched the scraps blowing away.

I never had the courage to confess."


"I can't watch television anymore.

It makes me sick all over again to see all

the body parts and blood."

Scan the page lightly. When something "pops out" or "tugs" on you, start writing immediately about whatever it reminds you of. Then ask yourself what difference it has made in your life.

"The doctor seems to know what he's doing, but I don't understand what he's saying. I guess I don't have to understand everything. If I can trust him, maybe the knot in my stomach will go away."

"Our car was speeding along Lake Shore Drive, three eight-year-old girls in the back and the two mothers in the front. Suddenly the back door swung open and one of the girls started to fall out. She was just barely holding on. I was afraid to try to grab her. Another girl grabbed her, but she fell out of the car anyway but wasn't hurt. My mother told my father later how ashamed she was of me for just sitting there and doing nothing."

"Christmas is supposed to be fun and loving and happy. But there is always trouble when the family gets together. Why does that happen?"

_____

_____

_____

_____

_____

_____

_____

_____

_____

_____

_____

_____

_____

_____

_____

_____

_____

_____

_____

_____

_____

Scan the page lightly. When something "pops out" or "tugs" on you, start writing immediately about whatever it reminds you of. Then ask yourself what difference it has made in your life.

# World War II

| | | |
|---|---|---|
| Air raid wardens | Blackouts | Censored letters and news |
| Cigarette shortages | Black market | Curfews |
| Rationing | Holocaust | Pearl Harbor |
| Gold stars in the window | Victory gardens | Walter Winchell |

_____

_____

_____

_____

_____

_____

_____

_____

_____

_____

_____

_____

Scan the page lightly. When something "pops out" or "tugs" on you, start writing immediately about whatever it reminds you of. Then ask yourself what difference it has made in your life.

"Flags everywhere. pro-peace, pro-war.

pro-liberal, pro-conservative.

Cars honking their horns in approval.

Angry words.

Songs of peace. Signs everywhere."

"The thing I hated most about gym was

waiting to be picked to be on a team.

I always got a pain in my chest waiting to be picked.

But I stood there trying to look like it didn't matter."

_____

_____

_____

_____

_____

_____

_____

_____

_____

_____

_____

_____

_____

_____

_____

_____

_____

_____

_____

_____

_____

_____

_____

_____

_____

_____

_____

_____

_____

_____

Scan the page lightly. When something "pops out" or "tugs" on you, start writing immediately about whatever it reminds you of. Then ask yourself what difference it has made in your life.

"I got my period in gym class. It was awful. So messy. The teacher helped me clean myself up and taught me how to use the Kotex. It felt so funny walking with that thing between my legs."

"I climbed up the ladder and started walking out on the high dive. It was so narrow. There was nothing to hold onto. My heart banged in my chest. I chickened out and turned to go back and saw someone waiting on the ladder, blocking the way, so I had to keep going. I took a few more steps—one out into the air. I hit the water with a slap and kept going to the bottom. It was deeper than I thought and I was short on air. I kicked like a madman to get to the top."

_____

_____

_____

Scan the page lightly. When something "pops out" or "tugs" on you, start writing immediately about whatever it reminds you of. Then ask yourself what difference it has made in your life.

"When I was little, Grandpa loved to take me to the movies, but he had to sit in the front row so he could hear. To me, the screen was filled with huge flat people and I was afraid that they would fall in my lap. The voices and music were so loud it felt like someone pounding nails into my ears. After the first time, I didn't want to go again, but I didn't want to hurt Grandpa's feelings either."

"At his graduation, my grandson comes over to me, gives me a hug and tells me he loves me."

Dear Julia,

You'll never guess who I saw at the reunion. Jake Stephens. Do you remember when I asked him to the girls' choice eighth grade dance and he said yes, but then his friends came over and sang gooey love songs under my window, and then he called the next day and cancelled? He's still cute, but bald and gutless. Besides, he's married. Dara

_____

_____

# Write Your Self Well Personal Healing Chart

Graph your responses each day after journaling, using 5 to indicate the most improvement and 1 the least.

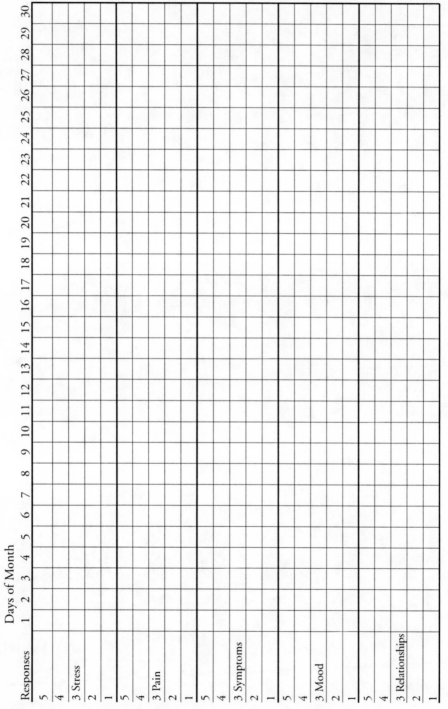

# Further Readings

1.  Adams, C. (1999). <u>A woman of wisdom: honoring &
    celebrating who you are</u>. Berkeley, CA: Celestial Arts.

2.  Adams, Kathleen. (1990). <u>Journal to the self: Twenty-
    two paths to personal growth</u>. New York: Warner
    Books, Inc.

3.  Adams, Kathleen. (1998). <u>The way of the journal: A
    journal therapy workbook for healing</u>. Baltimore,
    MD: The Sidran Press.

4.  Albert, S. Wittig. (1996). <u>Writing from life: Telling
    your soul's story: a journey of self-discovery for
    women</u>. New York: Jeremy P. Tarcher/Putnam,
    Penguin Putnam, Inc.

5.  Albom, M. (2003). <u>The five people you meet in
    heaven</u>. New York: Hyperion.

6.  Allen, R. (2003). <u>The playful way to knowing yourself</u>.
    New York: Houghton Mifflin.

7.  Ban Breathnach, S. (1996). <u>Simple abundance journal
    of gratitude</u>. New York: Warner Books.

8. Bateson, M. (1989). <u>Composing a life</u>. New York: Grove Press.

9. Bowers, S. C., & Norman, J. W. (1987). <u>A woman's journal: A step-by-step journey to recovery</u>. Asheville, NC: Appalachian Hall.

10. Cameron, J. & Collins, J. (2002). <u>Walking in this world: The practical art of creativity</u>. New York: Tarcher/Putnam, Penguin Putnam, Inc.

11. Capacchione, L. (2002). <u>The creative journal: The art of finding yourself</u>. Franklin Lakes, NJ: New Page Books, Division of the Career Press.

12. Charman, R. (1992). <u>At risk: Can the doctor-patient relationship survive in the high-tech world?</u> Dublin, NH: William L. Bauhan, Publisher.

13. Dass, R. (2000). <u>Still here: Embracing aging, changing, and dying</u>. New York: Riverhead Books/Penguin Putnam Inc.

14. Davis, M., Eshelman, E. & McKay, M. (2000). <u>The relaxation and stress reduction workbook</u>. Oakland, CA: New Harbinger Publications, Inc.

15. Dayringer, R. (1998). <u>The heart of pastoral counseling: Healing through relationship</u>. New York: Haworth Personal Press, Inc.

16. De Salvo, L. (1999). <u>Writing as a way of healing: How telling our stories transforms our lives</u>. Boston, MA: Beacon Press.

17. Gerteis, M., Edgman-Levitan, S., Daley, J., & Delbanco, T.L. (1993). <u>Through the patient's eyes: Understanding and promoting patient-centered care</u>. San Francisco: Jossey-Bass Publishers.

18. Greenspan, M. (2004). <u>Healing through the dark emotions: The wisdom of grief, fear, and despair</u>. Boston & London: Shambhala.

19. Gunther, J. (1949) <u>Death be not proud</u>. New York: Harper Perennial.

20. Hagan, K. L. (1988). Internal affairs: <u>A journal keeping workbook for self-intimacy</u>. Atlanta, GA: Escapadia Press.

21. Hardin, P. (1992) <u>What are you doing with the rest of your life? Choices in midlife.</u> San Rafael, CA: New World Library.

22. Heilbrun, C. (1998). <u>The last gift of time: Life beyond sixty</u>. New York: The Dial Press, Bantam Doubleday Dell Publishing Group, Inc.

23. Kaye, R. (1991). <u>Spinning straw into gold: Your emotional recovery from breast cancer</u>. New York: Fireside, Simon and Schuster.

24. Keel, Philipp. (1998). <u>All about me</u>. New York: Broadway Books.

25. Kessler, D. (1997). <u>The rights of the dying: A companion for life's final moments</u>. New York: HarperCollins Publishing, Inc.

26. Leder, D. (1997). <u>Spiritual passages: Embracing life's sacred journey</u>. New York: Jeremy P. Tarcher/Putnam.

27. Luke, H. (1987). <u>Old age: Journey into simplicity</u>. New York: Parabola Books.

28. Miller, D. (2003). <u>Your surviving spirit: A spiritual workbook for coping with trauma</u>. Oakland, CA: New Harbinger Publications, Inc.

29. Moore, N. & Komras, H. (1993). <u>Patient-focused healing: Integrating caring and curing in health care</u>. San Francisco: Jossey-Bass Publishers.

30. Paivio, A. (1971). <u>Imagery and verbal processes</u>. New York: Holt.

31. Rich, P. (1999). <u>The healing journey through grief: Your journal for reflection and recovery</u>. New York: John Wiley & Sons, Inc.

32. Rybarczyk, B. & Bellg, A. (1997). <u>Listening to life stories: A new approach to stress intervention in health care</u>. New York: Springer Publishing Company.

33. Sark. (1993). <u>Sark's journal and play! book: A place to dream while awake</u>. Berkeley, CA: Celestial Arts.

34. Schachter-Shalomi, Z. & Miller, R. (1995). <u>From age-ing to sage-ing: A profound new vision of growing older</u>. New York: Warner Books.

35. Segalove, I. & Velick. P. (1996). <u>List your self: Listmaking as the way to self-discovery: A provocative, probing and personal expedition into your mind, heart and soul</u>. Kansas City: Andrews and McMeel, A Universal Press Syndicate Co.

36. Sheehy, L. (2000). <u>I haven't talked about this before: The story of a family's journey into the world of cancer</u>. Winter Park, FL: Four Seasons Publishers, Inc.

37. Starkman, E. (1993). <u>Learning to sit in the silence: A journal of caretaking</u>. Watsonville, CA: Papier-Mache Press.

38. Zimmermann, S. (2002). <u>Writing to heal the soul: Transforming grief and loss through writing</u>. New York: Three Rivers Press.

# References

1.  Antoni, M.H. (1999). <u>Empirical studies of emotional disclosure in the face of stress: a progress report</u>. ADVANCES: The Journal of Mind/Body Medicine. 15: 163 – 165.

2.  Bachelard, G. (1960). <u>The poetics of reverie: Childhood, language and the cosmos</u>. Boston: Beacon Press.

3.  Bachelard, G. (1958). <u>The poetics of space: The classic look at how we experience intimate places</u>. Boston: Beacon Press.

4.  Dienstfrey, H. (1999). <u>Disclosure and health: an interview with James W. Pennebaker</u>. ADVANCES: The Journal of Mind/Body Medicine, 15, l6l – 170.

5.  Hunter, K. Montgomery (1991). <u>Doctors' stories: The narrative structure of medical knowledge</u>. Princeton, NJ: Princeton University Press.

6.  Jackins, H. (1978). <u>The human side of human beings: The theory of re-evaluation counseling</u>. Seattle, WA: Rational Island Publishers.

7.  Lepore, S. & Smyth, J. (2002). <u>The writing cure: How expressive writing promotes health and well-being</u>. Washington, D.C.: American Psychological Association.

8.  Litowitz, B. & Epstein, P. Eds. (1991). <u>Semiotic perspectives on clinical theory and practice: Medicine, neuropsychiatry and psychoanalysis</u>. Berlin, New York: Mouton de Gruyter.

9.  Lutgendorf, S. & Ullrich, P. (2002). <u>Something to write home about: Journaling can help after trauma</u>. Annals of Behavioral Medicine. August 19.

10. Paivio, A. (1971). <u>Imagery and verbal processes. Thought and image</u>. New York: Holt.

11. Pavio, A. (1990). <u>Mental Representations</u>. New York: Oxford University Press.

12. Pennebaker, J.W. (1999). <u>Inhibition, disclosure and health/response</u>. ADVANCES: The Journal of Mind/Body Medicine. 15, 193 – 195.

13. Pennebaker, J.W. (1997). <u>Opening up: The healing power of expressing emotions</u>. New York: The Guilford Press.

14. Pennebaker, J.W. (2002). <u>Emotion, disclosure & health</u>. Washington, D.C.: American Psychological Association.

15. Progoff, I. (1998). <u>At a journal workshop</u>. New York: J.P. Tarcher/Putnam.

16. Schultz, J. (1990). <u>Writing from start to finish: The 'story workshop' basic forms rhetoric-reader</u>. Concise Edition, Portsmouth, NH: Boynton/Cook, Heinemann.

17. Schultz, J. (1990). <u>The teacher's manual for writing start to finish: the story workshop manual</u>. Montclair, NJ: Boynton.

18. Schur, M. R. (1992). <u>The reading woman: A journal</u>. San Francisco: Pomegranate Artbooks.

19. Smyth, J. M. (1998). <u>Written emotional expression: Effect sizes, outcome types and moderating variables</u>. Journal of Consulting and Clinical Psychology. 66, 174 – 184.

20. Smyth, J., Stone, A., Hurewitz, A., & Kaell, A. (1999). <u>Effects of writing about stressful experiences on symptom reduction in patients with asthma or rheumatoid arthritis: A randomized trial</u>. Journal of the American Medical Association, 281: 1304 - 1309.

21. Smyth, J. (1999). <u>Written disclosure: Evidence, potential mechanism and potential treatment</u>. ADVANCES: The Journal of Mind-Body Medicine, 15, 161-195.

22. Spiegel, D., Bloom, J., Kraemer, H., & Gottheil, E. (1989). Effect of psychosocial treatment on survival of patients with metastatic breast cancer. Lancet 2: 888-891.

23. Vygotsky, L.S. (1972). Thought and language. Cambridge, MA: MIT.

24. Wilhelm, J. D., Baker, T. N. & Dube, J. (2001). Strategic reading. Portsmouth, NH: Heinemann.

# Resource Organizations

Having said all that you've said and written all that you've written, you may feel a need for additional resources and support. Journaling is a process of discovery—about yourself, about the past, about what you want in the future. Maybe you've unearthed an event that continues to be disturbing—something that affects you in a way you don't understand, that's upsetting, or continues to nag at you. Maybe writing about it simply isn't enough. What to do?

First, talk to your doctor or your therapist. He or she can guide you or recommend competent professionals who can help you sort out these issues.

In addition, we list a number of national resources, most with local or regional chapters or offices, that provide information about specific physical or emotional areas of concern. This is not an exhaustive list. We are all overwhelmed with the volumes of information available about healthcare, particularly on the Internet. People who are healthcare communications professionals helped compile our reference list from credible sources. We think you'll find it helpful.

## Resources:

**Association for Death Education and Counseling**
e-mail: info@adec.org
www.ADEC.org
342 North Main St.
West Hartford, CT 06117-2507
Phone: (860) 586-7503

Their goal is to enhance the ability of professionals and lay people to be better able to meet the needs of those with whom they work in death education and grief counseling.

**Federation of Families for Children's Mental Health**

e-mail: ffcmh@ffcmh.org

www.ffcmh.org

1101 King St., Suite 420

Alexandria, VA 22314

Phone: (706) 684-7710

An advocacy organization with 120 state offices that represents children, youth and families from diverse cultures and backgrounds.

**National Alliance for Mental Illness**

www.nami.org

Colonial Place Three

2107 Wilson Blvd., Suite 300

Arlington, VA 22201-3042

Phone: 800-950-NAMI (6264)

Founded in 1979, they work to achieve equitable services and treatment for more than 15 million Americans. They are dedicated to the eradication of mental illness and to the improvement of the quality of life of all those whose lives are affected by these diseases.

## National Mental Health Association

www.nmha.org

2001 N. Beauregard St., 12<sup>th</sup> Floor

Alexandria, VA 22311

Phone: (703) 684-7722 or 800-969-NMHA (6642)

TTY Line: 800-433-5959

The oldest and largest nonprofit organization of its kind with 340 affiliates. Addresses all aspects of mental health and mental illness.

## National Center for Complementary and Alternative Medicine

www.nccam.nih.gov/health/decisions

NCCAM Clearinghouse

P.O. Box 7923

Gaithersburg, MD 20898-7923

Phone: 888-644-6226

Assists you in making decisions about your health—whether to use complementary and alternative medicine (CAM). It includes frequently asked questions, issues to consider, and a list of sources for further information. The site offers related topics in Spanish and a medical dictionary. Topics are discussed by treatment or therapy and by disease or condition.

**Alcoholics Anonymous**

www.aa.org

Grand Central Station

P.O. Box 459

New York, New York 10163

Located throughout the U.S., AA is a fellowship of men and women who share experience, strength and hope with each other that they may solve their common problem and help others recover from alcoholism. Consult your local telephone book for chapters in your area.

**The National Institute on Aging**

www.nia.nih.gov

Bldg. 31, Room 5C27

31 Center Drive, MSC 2292

Bethesda, MD 20892

Phone: (301) 496-1752

Federal government site with the latest information and research on aging and resources to contact. Covers all diseases associated with aging.

**Alzheimer's Association and Related Disorders, Inc**

www.alzassoc.org

225 North Michigan Ave., Suite 1700

Chicago, IL 60601

Phone: 800-272-3900

A leader in research, support and fund raising with local chapters across the country and a network of advocates.

**American Stroke Association**

Division of American Heart Association

www.strokeassociation.org

National Center

7272 Greenville Ave.

Dallas, TX 75231

Phone: 1-888-4STROKE

Site includes programs, Heart Stroke Encyclopedia of information, news, and fund raising opportunities.

## National Women's Health Information Center

www.4woman.gov

8550 Arlington Blvd., Suite 300

Fairfax VA, 22031

Phone: 800-994-WOMAN (9662)

Federal government site for free, reliable information on 800 women's health topics.

## American Diabetes Association

www.diabetes.org

1701 North Beauregard St.

Alexandria, VA 22311

Phone: 1-800-DIABETES (342-2383)

Nonprofit health organization offers research, information and advocacy. Founded in 1940, it conducts programs in all 50 states and the District of Columbia, reaching more than 800 communities.

eHealthcare Strategy & Trends
Leadership Award Winners 2003
Best Health/Healthcare Content

## Hospital Centers of Excellence:

The Cleveland Clinic Heart Center. clevelandclinic.org/heart-center

Cancer Treatment Centers of America, IL. cancercenter.com

University of Texas health Science Center at Houston. health-leader.uthouston.edu

The Cleveland Clinic Dept. of Gastroenterology & Hematology. clevelandclinic.org/gastro

The Cleveland Clinic Neuroscience Center. clevelandclinic.org/neuroscience

## HMO/PPO/Other Insurers:

Blue Cross & Blue Shield of Minnesota. blueprint.blue-crossmn.com

Humana Inc., KY. humana.com

Independence Blue Cross, PA. site65.com/health65

Horizon Blue Cross Blue Shield of New Jersey. horizon-bcb-snj.com

Anthem, Inc., IN. home.anthemhealth.com

**Consumer General Health Sites:**
Aetna InteliHealth Inc., PA. intelihealth.com

Mayo Clinic, MN. mayoclinic.com

HealthVision/VHA Inc., TX. laurushealth.com

Choice Media, TX. healthcentral.com

Advance PCS, TX. buildingbetterhealth.com

BreastCenter.org, PA. breastcancer.org

Body1 Inc., MA. heart1.com

CenterWatch, MA. centerwatch.com

AACC, DC. labtestsonline.org

Humana Military Healthcare Services, KY. humana-military.com

Centers for Medicare & Medicaid Services, MD. medicare.gov

# Ina Albert, APR, APRP

Ina Albert has been a healthcare communications professional, trainer and workshop leader for more than 30 years. She developed and facilitated workshops and conducted trainings on interpersonal communications to improve patient satisfaction and staff relations and retention at major hospitals in New Jersey, Florida and Illinois. For the past eleven years, she has directed customer service and patient satisfaction programs for a healthcare network in Illinois.

Ms. Albert has been a healthcare communications consultant for psychiatric hospitals, experiential therapists, alternative practices, nursing homes, and behavioral health organizations. She developed and facilitated workshops for healthcare providers, clinical staff, business groups and individuals in vision management and interpersonal communication skills. More recently, she has been leading Life Transition and Vital Aging workshops for older adults.

Ms. Albert is a certified seminar leader for Spiritual Eldering Institute in Boulder, CO, and for Private Paths, Common Ground, a life transitions workshop created through Midway Center for Creative Imagination in Washington, D.C.

In addition to her work in healthcare communications, she has directed healthcare marketing and public relations programs and has written numerous articles on healthcare communications, patient relations and alternative medicine for major health care publications including <u>Conscious Choice</u> and <u>Strategic Healthcare Marketing Newsletter</u>. Ms. Albert also has published several short stories in <u>Chicago Parent Magazine</u> and <u>Hudson Valley Magazine</u>.

A graduate of Brandeis University in Waltham, MA, she has completed graduate studies in Foundations of Holistic Health at De Paul University in Chicago.

# Zoe Keithley, MATW

Ms. Keithley, who has a Master of Arts in the Teaching of Writing, is a master teacher and director in the renowned Story Workshop® at Columbia College, Chicago, where she taught fiction for fifteen years. In addition, she served as writing workshop director and archivist for *Tell Your Story Project*, a celebration of Chicago's sesquicentennial. She is now living, teaching and writing in Northern California.

Her training in fiction writing at Columbia College, Chicago, and fifteen years on the fiction writing staff there give her a deep writing stratum that is both theoretical and practical. More recently, she has been privately coaching fiction and non-fiction writers. Ms. Keithley inspired creativity and imagination among students in elementary and high school classes, in college and graduate students and among adult learners.

Ms. Keithley was a writing specialist for Northeastern Illinois University and Chicago Public Schools. She is the author of "Image and Reading," a chapter in a collection on reading edited by specialist Jeffrey Wilhelm.

Since 1983, Ms. Keithley has been publishing fiction, non-fiction and poetry in national magazines and through Columbia College and Northeastern Illinois University. Her artistic performances, including prose readings, poetry and music, have been held throughout the Chicagoland area over the past several years.

A prize-winning author in fiction and poetry, she was a finalist in the 2001 Zoetrope All-Story Competition, an Illinois Arts Council Fellow (1997), and a finalist in American Fiction, V.9, 1997. She holds a number of other awards as well and is published in prose, including contributing breakthrough research on "Voice" in the Journal of Basic Writing (1992), Crain's Chicago Business (1987) and Conscious Choice (1999).

She is a graduate of Trinity College in Washington, D.C and Columbia College, Chicago.

# Interactive Presentations and Workshops

If you enjoyed this book, the programs listed here might be of interest to you. Ina Albert and Zoe Keithley are experienced teachers and facilitators, working with groups and organizations across the country to demonstrate the healing benefits of journaling.

• **Write Your Self Well** – This interactive journaling workshop helps patients get in touch with the stresses that contribute to their suffering and tap into their healing strengths. Ina and Zoe have developed a unique journaling process that makes it easy and fun to explore important issues and experiences in your life, to write about them and put yourself on the road to health. The workshop is based on 20-plus years of clinical research that demonstrate the positive benefits of expressive writing.

• **Write Your Relationships Well** – A couples workshop that uses interactive journaling as a tool for understanding one another. The goal of the experiential exercises is to build a family vision by identifying shared social and spiritual values while designing your family culture. Led by Ina Albert and her husband, Rabbi Allen Secher, a nationally recognized leader and counselor in assisting interfaith partners integrate their separate heritages with each other and their families.

• **Write Your Life Well** – Our stories are our legacies. Older adults explore their life experiences through journaling and discover the positive effect expressive writing has on their health and on relationships in the family and community. This inspiring intergenerational program, led by Ina Albert, is available as an interactive presentation or workshop for seniors and healthcare, civic, religious organizations and schools.

• **Vital Aging** – This one-day workshop explores the 21st century senior's expanded role as longevity increases. No previous generation has lived longer, been healthier, wealthier or more powerful. The program offers a framework for enjoying these benefits by creating positive change, a healthy lifestyle and exciting growth through life's transitions experienced in later years. Ina Albert presents a roadmap to use these benefits to live with vitality.

- **Private Paths, Common Ground** – An Adult Rite of Passage. Gain a new perspective on aging. Together with your fellow workshop participants, step into a place of self-discovery and self-expression and rediscover the creativity and imagination that can guide you through life transitions and help you create your vision for the future. A certified trainer in this groundbreaking experiential work, Ina Albert asks that you take time to stop and step out of your daily routine to assess where you are and where you are going.

- **Age-ing to Sage-ing'** – A Profound New Vision of Growing Older- In this Age of Aging, everyone needs to learn how to grow older with dignity, wisdom and a sense of value as a human being. This workshop teaches participants how to live consciously and plan for the end of life as a natural part of the aging process. Ina Albert is a certified seminar leader for the Spiritual Eldering Institute, dedicated to the work of Zalman Schachter-Shalomi, theologian, philosopher, teacher, rabbi, and creator of this work.

Communication Coaching for Healthcare
Professionals

- **The Space in Between** – How to Be Good Medicine-
Explore how healthy communication can become good
therapy for both patients and health care providers.
Improve team performance, patient satisfaction and
relationships with colleagues by learning to use the
principles of energy communication that are a crucial to
patient care and a healing environment. Facilitated by Ina
Albert, this is a valuable introductory program to
customer service program or staff training for schools,
hospitals and healthcare organizations.

For information on any of these programs, call
Ina Albert Associates, LLC, (406) 863-2333,
e-mail writeforhealth@aol.com, or visit our
web site, www.writeyourself.com.